The Slow Goodbye: D......, ...
with Dementia

This book is an anthology of short blogs written by a daughter and granddaughter while they make hard choices for their loved one, as she moves through the stages of dementia. Some of the blogs are very personal, but they are written from the heart. We can only hope that others that faced with this situation can find some comfort from this and know that they are not alone.

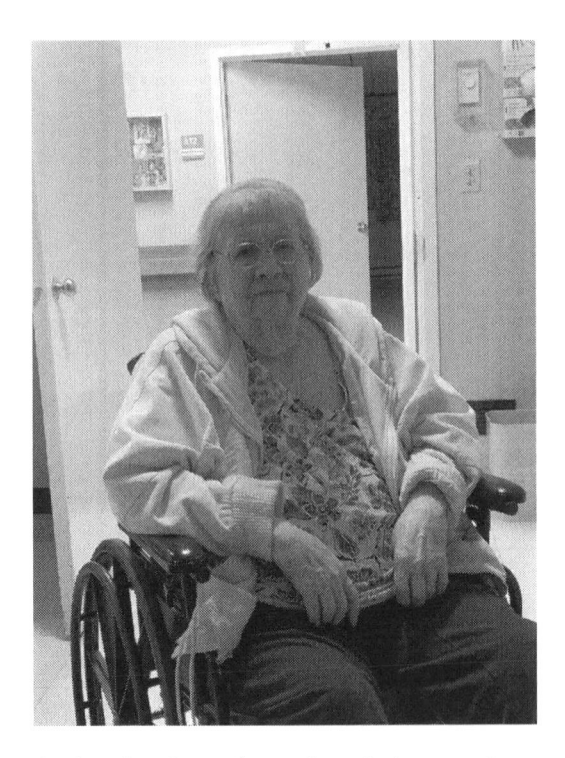

Dedicated to the most loving daughter, sister, sister-in-law, mother, grandmother, & great grandmother I know. LOVE YOY MA

MANY RESOURCES TO HELP WHEN DEALING WITH DEMENTIA

WHY THE SLOW GOODBYE?

STAGES OF DEMENTIA

TALKING TO YOUR LOVED ONE WITH DEMENTIA

HAVING A MEANINGFUL CONVERSATION WITH A LOVE ONE

THE SLOW GOODBYE

DON'T ASK

WHAT UNDERSTANDING CAN MEAN

CAREGIVER STRESS - ALL CAREGIVERS HAVE IT.

ONE OF THE HARDEST REALIZATIONS I'VE EVER HAD

ROADMAPS FOR OUR LOVE ONES

AS THE FINAL GLIMMER OF MY MOM DWINDLES AWAY:

DIFFICULT PAPERWORK

DADDY'S LITTLE GIRL TO MOM'S CARETAKER

WOULD YOU WANT TO KNOW IF YOU MAY INHERIT DEMENTIA?

IS THE GREATEST GIFT LOVE, TIME OR BOTH?

LETTING IT GO

BE BRAVE AND GO AWAY ALONE FOR SELF-CARE

KNOWLEDGE IS POWER: TESTING FOR DEMENTIA

Many resources to help when dealing with Dementia

AlzConnected.org There are many resources to help. I have found discussion board to have a wealth of knowledge. I have joined the caregiver's forum. I have a few post from my blogs there. We have some great conversions. This is one post I made that put a smile on my face. This shows we are not alone, and even if we do not know each other, we can help each other.

"This is such a timely post for me as well - thank you for sharing. I've been holding on to the signed DNR form, afraid to give it to my mom's new assisted living facility, because the weight of making that kind of decision for another person, feels too great. I will turn the form in today because I know in my heart that my mom wouldn't want any extraordinary measures to be taken. We watched it happen to my grandmother who also had Alzheimer's and we all said never again. This is the supportive nudge that I needed to do the right thing."

Why the Slow Goodbye?

Why this book is titled the Slow Goodbye? If you've ever had someone in your life that had dementia you know that it can go on for years. My mom has had dementia for more than 10 years. There are stages that she goes through, and with every stage that it takes on, that person you loved away gets further away from you.

When you get to the latest stages, the person you once knew is gone. They are still there physically, but they cannot do the activities that they once did. They cannot go trips with you, they cannot go to dinner with you, and they cannot watch the grandkids for you.

"The Slow Goodbye" means that each day, you lose just a little bit more of that person. "The Slow Goodbye" is knowing that the end is soon, but it could take years. You experience something called anticipatory grief. Meaning - you are grieving the loss of the person before they pass. Each day, when you say goodbye, you never know if it may be the last.

Stages of Dementia

Mild Dementia

In this early stage of dementia, an individual can still function rather independently, and often is still able to drive and maintain a social life. In the very early stage of dementia, symptoms that are seen may be attributed to the normal process of aging.

Moderate Dementia

In this middle stage of dementia, which in most cases is the longest stage of the disease, brain damage is extensive enough that a person has trouble expressing their thoughts, performing daily tasks, and has more severe memory issues than in the earlier stage

Severe Dementia

In late stage dementia, also known as advanced dementia, individuals have significant issues with communication, often using only words or expressions. At the very end, they may not verbally communicate at all.

Source: https://www.dementiacarecentral.com/aboutdementia/facts/stages/

Talking to your loved one with dementia

Not only does my mom have dementia, but my mother-in-law also had a form of dementia. They were two different types, however. My mother-in-law's dementia did not make her as forgetful, but instead as she believed in situations that were not really true. Going back to my golden rules in my last post I never argued or disagreed with her. Instead, I listened to her stories and, when appropriate, had a good laugh with her. It was funny because for the first 20 years our relationship was not the best. The impression I got was that I was the one that took their only son away from them. As time passed, and illness came about, I would often go into Boston by myself to see her and to, again, listen and not disagree with her stories. She passed 4 years ago, but I was truly blessed to have the time spent with her, and in the end, I do believed that she loved me as I loved her.

So, when dealing with a loved one with dementia, try to make the visit enjoyable for both of you. I know it can be hard at times, especially after working 8+ hrs. Meeting after meeting. Take the time, however, to leave the pressures of life and job at the door. What I do is listen to my favorite band (Coldplay) before I go in from work, it always lifts my spirits and put me in good frame of mind.

LOVE YOU MOM!!!!!

Having a meaningful conversation with a love one

I have been asked many times how to have a conversation with a loved one with Dementia. They always ask the same question over and over again. This is what I have learned over the past few years: Always answer the question, never say "I already answered that question" Instead, agree with them, because does it really matter, don't argue with them if they have a fact wrong,

1. Don't try to reason with them, instead divert the conversion to something they like, for me it is always hockey.

2. Don't lecture them on useless facts, instead reassure the feelings they are having

3 Never ever ask them if they remember, you already know the answer, instead tell them a story about what happened at that event.

4. Don't say I told you, instead repeat and add a new tidbit.

5 Don't say "you can't". Instead encourage what they can do.

6. Never be condescending, remember - they are your mother, father, or loved one. Instead encourage them to express themselves

Time is something we do not have enough of. Time is something that can make you feel "crazy", especially when you're waiting for something special. Time can go by so fast that it takes your breath away. Time can also go so slow that it's very painful. We wish for more time with love ones, we hate wasting time.

As for Mom with dementia, time has no tangible meaning to her, but in reality, time has done a great deal of good for her in the past few weeks. Time has helped my Mom make new friends at her new residence, and it has helped her be happier than I have seen her in years. Time has healed her wounds. Time has made a scary place for her into a lovely, social environment for her and for her family. Time has helped me appreciate my Mom now - not the Mom I had before dementia.

This is something that I have been struggling with since I made the decision to move her into a nursing home. When dementia first started affecting her, I found myself missing the mother I knew from 10, 20, 30 years prior. Time healed me also, however. Spending quality time with my Mom made me love her in different way, a way that was more loving and caregiving. I know now that it is my time to take care of her, like she did for me. With whatever time I get to spend with her in these later stages of life will always be the best TIME of my life.

The Slow Goodbye

The stress of caring for a loved one with dementia can be overwhelming. For the past few months, that has been my case. It's not that my mom is needing more care, it's the fact that her dementia is moving toward its final stages. Not that any doctor has told us that, it is from watching her closely and noting some different behaviors.

My Mom has been constantly asking why my Dad is not coming to see her and what is he is doing. He passed 24 and a half years ago, and Mom knew this up until the past few months. She also asks for her brother, who he passed 10 years ago.

What I was told in a support group for dementia caregivers, which I highly recommend, is that she currently thinks of herself at a certain age, perhaps her mid 50's, when my Dad and Uncle were alive. Before I attended the group, I was telling her that Dad is no longer with us. This caused incredible sadness to come over her daily. That was the wrong thing to do. Their suggested is to tell a "fiblet" or re-direct her thoughts somewhere else, which worked. No one told me the profound sadness I would have to see her slipping away, and myself reliving the death of my Dad & Uncle.

Another suggestion made was that when dementia patience are preparing for the end, they will ask about love ones that are gone. They may even say that they saw them. They will ask to go home, and when you ask them which home, they often say their childhood home. This is what is going on now, for my Mom. When asked which home, she replies her childhood home to see her Mom & Dad. This information is the most stressful for me. Knowing this is sometimes too much to handle. According to Lisa Williams, this process is sometimes called "Grieving before a Death", or Anticipatory Grief.

"This occurs when you are grieving before a loved one has passed. Symptoms of anticipatory grief are– sadness, anger, isolation, forgetfulness, and depression. When we know a death is imminent our bodies are often in a state of hyper-alertness – we panic whenever the phone rings, an ambulance must be called, or when our loved one deteriorates. This can become mentally and physically exhausting."

It is like they are looking into my life. As they say, knowledge is power, and I intend to gather knowledge and guidance on dealing with these issues. There is a podcast called "Anticipatory Grief", for when grief begins before a loss or death. It is very informative and helpful. I suggest you seek out an understanding support team, a friend, therapist, support group all can help, even all three. It is hard to talk about, so find people that will listen. People say "well at least she is alive." They do not understand. Yes, she is physically here with me, but the Mother I have loved all my life, and still do, is gone forever. That my friends is the "Slow goodbye of dementia"

Don't Ask

Do not ask me to remember,

Don't try to make me understand,

Let me rest and know you're with me,

Kiss my cheek and hold my hand.

I'm confused beyond your concept,

I am sad and sick and lost.

All I know is that I need you

To be with me at all cost.

Do not lose your patience with me,

Do not scold or curse or cry.

I can't help the way I'm acting,

Can't be different though I try.

Just remember that I need you,

That the best of me is gone,

Please don't fail to stand beside me,

Love me 'til my life is done.

What Understanding can mean

Although we all know the meaning of the word, it touches us in different ways.

1. Understand that you need to take care of yourself while moving through life with a parent that has dementia. This has been hard for me, but quickly, I've realized that I cannot put my life on hold for ten years. Yes, I travel to Europe at times with my daughter. I find the mother-daughter trips to be ones that I will hold dear to my heart forever. I wish I could have done this with my Mom. It's helpful to have a backup plan, just in case I get the "Call" that my Mom is sick (or worse). I run over the scenarios over and over again in my mind. I make sure that I have all the phone numbers for flights back, I think of who I would call first in the event of an emergency, and I make sure my phone that has international plan is with me at all times. If I go on an all day tour, I must make extra preparations. This isn't overreacting, this is necessary preparation for me to be simultaneously responsible and have a good time.

2. Understand that the little things you can do to make your loved one feel better. Every Sunday, when I can, I bring my Mom a coffee and a muffin from Dunkin. We enjoy that time, and she always says "Wow this muffin is so fresh!" I also run down to her nursing home, when I can, before the Boston Bruins play to put the game on. My mom is the biggest hockey Fan I know. Hence my love for hockey, and why I played many years as a goalie. My mom, sitting in the heated area at Skate 3, watched my every game. I try to engage her with the sport when I can, as much as I can. There are times I can't, and that's

okay. I used to beat myself up about this, the guilt was overwhelming. I'm working on realizing that sometimes I just can't be there on Sunday or when the Bruins play.

3. Understand that your love ones will forget the event, and that's okay. Keep it up. The next day, after I put the Hockey game on for her, she asked me when the Bruins start their season. I explained to her that I put it on for her last night. I saw the confused look on her face. I'm learning to re-direct my comments. My daughter was able to take an hour of rehabilitation training for dementia patients though her job. She explained that dementia patients will forget the event but will not forget the emotion. For example, my mom forgot that she watched the game the next day, but she remembered the great feeling of watching the Bruins again. Understanding can help you through dealing with the uncharted territory of dementia.

Caregiver Stress - all caregivers have it.

As I mentioned, I plan on gaining more knowledge about dementia by way of research. I also want to learn how to take care of myself while moving through this disease with my Mom. My daughter sent me some information that I would like to share with you all. I can say that over the past 10 years, myself or a family member have, at some point, identified with every one of these symptoms. Under each symptom I will add in how it affected me, and some helpful hints on how to deal with the symptom.

Denial: About the disease and its effect on the person who has been diagnosed. I said to myself: Oh she will get better, or it is just old age. I was in denial for a long time, but when I faced it, I was able to help my mom in a more caring loving, and understand way. Get your loved one tested as soon as possible.

Anger: At the person with Alzheimer's or frustration that they can't do the things they used to be able to do. I never had this, but family members did. I would explain to the family member that this is how the disease is, and that you have to be understanding. I tried to listen to their concerns, but I grew frustrated at the constant phone calls saying, "Ma just asked me again when the Bruins are on." My anger was not with my Mom, but with family members.

Social withdrawal: Withdrawal from friends and activities that used to make you feel good. This is something that you do, but really don't know that you are doing this. In my previous blog, I said that you need to have a plan in your head for "the call" when socializing. I always do. Some days, it changes based on recent events and how far I'm traveling, but I always know what I will do if the nursing home calls me.

Anxiety: About the future and facing another day. This was at its highest last summer, when there was nothing we could do but move Mom into a nursing home for dementia patients. There were many sleepiness nights, as the guilt was overwhelming. With good friends, however, and supportive family, I'm now in the place where I believe this is the best for my mom.

Depression: It breaks your spirit and affects your ability to cope. This is ongoing for me, and there are many reasons to be depressed. The fact my Mom is not the same person she was 10 years ago is a huge trigger for me. When a friend talks about doing an activity with their Mom, one that I cannot do anymore with her, it makes me sad. Sometimes, I'm just sad that she is going through this, and there is absolute nothing you can do about it.

Exhaustion: It makes it nearly impossible to complete necessary daily tasks. I'm too busy for sleeplessness caused by a never-ending list of concerns, it makes me unnecessarily tired. For me, it is waking up at 3, 4 and 5 am checking my phone. It is the endless, wondering if I did not see her that day, is she ok, and is my Mom sick.

Irritability: It may leads to moodiness and triggers negative responses and actions. Leave me alone! I cannot tell you how many times I say this, or just remove myself from others so I can be alone. I was just recently asked, "Why were you so irritable, the other day?" If only others knew what goes through my head each day, you would be irritable, too. I cannot always put on the happy face for others, there are times I just need to be sad or even a bitch. My close friends understand that but others, I just blow it off.

Health problems: This can begin to take a mental and physical toll. Hell yes, this is so true. So take care of yourself mentally. This may look like having a close friend to talk to, a support group, or a therapist. I still find it hard to talk to people about how this is affecting me because I do not want to bother them, or come across as needy. We all need help along the way, however.

To quote my dorm song from the old college days (Friends from Elton John) "With a friend at hand you will see the light if your friends are there, then everything's all right"

So in the long and short of things, TAKE CARE OF YOURSELF SO YOU CAN BE THE BEST FOR YOUR LOVE ONE.

Source: https://www.alz.org/help-support/caregiving/caregiver-health/

One of the hardest Realizations I've ever had

"Courage isn't having the strength to go on - it is going on when you don't have strength."

Warning: this is extremely personal, but I hope it helps others.

Recently, during a therapy session, I was asked the question that has been going through my head over and over again, but would never say out loud. The question hurts deeply, and once admitted to, is hard to get past. Once the cat is out of the bag, you cannot put back in. It can, and will, haunt me now and most likely forever.

The question that was posed to me, in such a matter of fact way, almost like she knew the answer before I could say it, was: "Do you wish that your Mom would pass away?" Wow, it shocked me to my core. I started to tear up right away, for two reasons. For even the thought of not having my Mom here, and the honest answer is, yes, I do think that. I took a breath and said, "I know in this setting I have to be honest or it will not help me, so, yes, I sometimes think that." While the tears were flowing, I said I can't be that selfish and uncaring, so I try to stop. I also said that I had a very close friend in ICU, and would pray that god would heal her and take my Mom instead. How could I ever think this, when I know that I love my Mom so much? I was told that this thinking is very normal for caregivers, and these feelings are to be expected. I understand this concept logically, but emotionally, I cannot get past it. There is much more work to be done for me. I can say, however, that I have been beating myself up over this for a long time. I asked myself, "how can I even think this, what kind of daughter am I?" I try to push my feelings down and put up a facade for everyone. I try to be the person people expect me to be, the funny one, the one that will help anyone at any time, the one that has all the answers, but in reality, I don't always have the answers. I don't have the answer to my life's burning questions: Why does my Mom have dementia? When will all this end? How can I help both my Mom and myself?

I push through by burying myself in my work and my volunteer activity. I find myself thinking that if my mind is occupied with other thoughts, then I will not think about this or the fact my Mom is suffering from dementia. That is a temporary fix, however. For example, I put my headphones on, then shut the world out, remove myself from everyone around me, but that does not work. I am alone with my thoughts. Again, there is so much more work to be done. All I can say is that, if you are having these feelings, YOU ARE NOT ALONE! You cannot fix your feeling ALONE, get help from any sources you have available to you.

Roadmaps for our love ones

In my professional life, I have road maps for projects. There are deadlines, milestones to achieve, and dates to meet. With caring for a love one with dementia, there is no such road map. Yes, there are stages, but not every person fits into a schedule.

Realizing this can be very difficult. You want to fit that round peg into the square hole to be able to adjust and prepare for what comes next. Sadly, however, that is not the case. For me, it is a constant monitoring of my Mom's actions and reactions. Lately, my Mom has forgotten names of children and their spouses. Which, if you were to look at the stages, this would be stage 6-7.

What do I do? How can I help my mother? This is the big question to which there is not much of an answer. What I can do is, with all the love in my heart, help her remember close family members. I won't make her feel guilty for not remembering. With love and patience, I will tell her "oh you forget…" and then remind her of an event with that person. At that moment, she may remember, but as I have noticed, she will ask again and forget - again. PATIENCE is the key here. Remember also that this is not a game, do not go into a visit and play "Let's see what Mom remembers today". Go with the mindset that you're going to have a great day with Mom, and when she is having a hard time remembering a person, guide her towards an event that she will fondly remember. There is no road map for this, however, I find it best to use the road map in your heart that only you know, and that will make your loved one happy.

Another casualty of not having a road map is that I find myself agonizing over this after my visits. I continue to beat myself up for not being a better daughter to my Mom. Why can't I help her get better? Why can't I let myself enjoy my time when I'm not with her? Why do I have many, many sleepiness nights worried that something happen to her?

Not only is there no road map for the progression of dementia patients, but there is also no road maps for caregivers. I have been told over and over again, "give yourself a break", "you are doing your best", and "you need to take care of yourself also". I know this, but it is very hard. I'm a commitment-driven person, I have committed to being there for my Mom since my dad past 24 years ago. Caring for myself isn't going to happen overnight, and it may never happen. I can work on the small things, like when I'm at an event, I can have a good time and keep telling myself that I'm allowed to have a good time.

While there are no road maps for our loved ones' awful disease, and no road maps for us caregivers, we need to understand that, in life, there are also no road maps. There are winding roads, road blocks, and road closures for all of us. Enjoy the ride, love the person you are taking care of, but most of all love yourself.

Stages of Dementia

https://www.alzheimers.net/stages-of-alzheimers-disease/

As the final glimmer of my mom dwindles away:

For the longest time, I always said "At least she recognizes me and the rest of her family." Well, that is going away more and more every day. This is the hardest symptom of dementia to deal with for me. You can see in their faces they are trying to remember yours from pictures, but, sadly, they cannot recall your face at that moment. You see this when they are confused when you arrive for your visit, not knowing who or why you are there.

This is what has happened to me over the past few weeks. I showed my mom a picture of a family member and she had no idea who they were, even when given clues still did not know them. Finally, after telling her their name, she seemed to recall. She even said, "how did I forget that?" Then, my daughter went to see Mom. At first, she was excited to see someone else, but after a few minutes, Mom was confused as to who she was talking to. This only lasted for a few moments, but the signs were there. Then the next day, I went for my visit. Normally, I go to the activities room, tap her on the shoulder, and I get a "Hi Karen how are you, how is everyone in the family?" This time, however, she asked me where I was taking her, and where she was going. It was like she did not know me and why I was there. This lasted only for a few moments, but the signs were there.

What can I do? I don't know right now, but what I know for sure is that I have to be patient and understanding. These are two things that if you know me, you know are not in my temperament much. This terrible, terrible dementia has taught me to be more patient and understanding. As it is heart-wrenching to discover her new symptoms, but I will approach it with more patience, understanding and LOVE. At the end of the day, love is the only thing that will help. The love of my family and friends that support and listen to me, and the LOVE of the woman that raised me to be patience, understanding, and a loving person.

Love ya MA.

Difficult Paperwork

Recently, I had a meeting with my Mom's case manager. During that meeting, the question that I never wanted to hear was posed to me. They said, "Your mom does not have a DNR (Do not resuscitate) order." My reply? I said that I know, and asked them why they brought it up. They said, at her advanced age, and with her stage of dementia, that it is the compassionate thing to do. Not to mention, this heavy conversion took place the day before Thanksgiving, which is the day we give thanks for our family and our many blessings.

I know what a "DNR" entails, but I did not know the extent that the orders go into. I did some research, as well as some soul searching. The complete form is called MOLST stands for Massachusetts Medical Orders for Life Sustaining Treatment. I talked to family and friends and was told that it is the compassionate thing to do. As long as it's the nice thing to do, it is also the hardest.

I then started asking questions almost telepathically to children who had signed this order for their parents. We're bonded almost cosmically. "How do you get your mindset past this road block? How to you sit there and watch your love one pass along when they get so ill that they need to be on a breathing machine? How can you claim to be a loving daughter and sign such papers?"

I don't have the answers, but I do know that I watched both my uncle and aunt slip away from me while I was sitting there holding their hands, all within 30 days of each other. At that time, I knew it was the compassionate thing we could have done. I also see other patients in my Mom's ward, that have gotten sick, been kept alive and now cannot feed themselves, cannot talk. Basically, their quality of life has left them.

I know that I don't want that for my mom. Is this selfish of me? I don't know, but I want my mom's quality of life be as good as it can be, she can still enjoy music, being with family (In small groups), and of course the Bruins.

So, on Thanksgiving I gave myself a break from all this, and enjoyed my time with my Mom. I counted my blessing to have three generations of Andres-Vergakes women in the same room. Today is other day, and yes I signed the paper, and will have to make peace with it, because it is the compassionate thing to do, even though it does not feel like that now.

This is just my opinion, and the place I'm at with my Mom. Everyone's choice is different and may not agree with me. Until you are faced with this question, you will never know the pain a health proxy goes through when faced with unspeakable decisions to make.

LOVE YA MA

Daddy's Little Girl to Mom's Caretaker

When I was younger, I was Daddy's girl. My dad could not start his car without me running out to ask him where he was going, and if I could come. I went to every softball game that he played in, and he was at every one of my softball, basketball and hockey games. He was always my biggest cheerleader. He taught me how to drive, he called the dean of students when I was caught with beer at college, and even payed the school for ice cream "we" stole from the dining hall. I called him every day. When he was struck with cancer in January 1994, I drove him to the VA in Boston, and went to see him every day until he passed that June. In a nutshell - he was the first man I truly loved.

On that day, when my world came crashing down, I became my mother's caregiver and have been since. She was only 64 at the time, and she did not have dementia yet. My Dad, however, did everything for her, so she was lost and did not know where to turn. At that point in my life, I was only married for 9 years. We had just bought our first home, and were going through some infertility issues. I was not ready to become my mother's caretaker. I just wanted to make her feel safe and secure. One night my Dad came to me in a dream, and very gently asked me to take care of my Mom. He said that she needed my loving care. He said that he was very proud of me and he knew I could do it. As a daughter that always did what my Dad wanted me to do, and did not want to disappoint him, I then became the best caregiver my mother could have ever wanted.

In the beginning, it only entailed having a joint checking account and making sure she was ok. A year later we had our first and only child. When she was born, she had my Dad's smile, and I know his spirit lives in her. We baptized her in the same church that we had my Dad's last goodbye in, it was a circle of life. My mom was serving as my mom, but she also she helped with our child. We went everywhere together, the three of us. My mom was a very engaged grandmother. I fondly remember her going to grandparent's day at my daughter's school.

As the years passed, I noticed that my mom would forget more and more. This was the start of dementia. The dementia got worse after she had kidney failure. At that point, I was doing more for her: setting up home care, meeting with doctors, explaining to her what was going with her health issues. I then became her full time caretaker.

Now, not only was I her caretaker, I was also her health proxy, making all the hard choices for her. I took on this role with all the love and gentleness that both my Dad and Mom showed me when I was growing up. Being a caretaker is hard work and can be very stressful. The fact that I know that my Mom is safe and secure, however, and that I am making all the right choices for her, is very rewarding as a daughter.

My advice? Be prepared to make those hard choices and to research everything when it comes to health care and financial options. Most importantly, find a support system in either family, friends, support groups or all three. Always remember - you are not alone in this role.

As my Dad asked me to do so many years ago, I am still my mom's caretaker and her biggest supporter. I know my Dad is proud of me and is guiding me through the rough waters of taking care of my Mom.

Would you want to know if you may inherit dementia?

One morning, I was just trying to mind my own business and reading through my endless emails, and a co-worker says to me, "Hey, did you hear that there is a gene you can be tested for to see if you may get dementia?" I said no, in a tone that would encourage them to leave me be. I can't let anything go when it comes to dementia, so I looked more into it. At that point, my thoughts were all over the place. I asked myself: do I read about this more, or do I stick my head in the sand and go through life as normal? If you know me, and as I have been told many times, I'm kind of a pain in the ass. I dig and dig until I get the answers I want or at least just an answer. So, I dug around and got my answers.

Here's a quick background of my family history of dementia. My mom, my maternal grandmother, and two uncles on my Dad's side all had/have a form of dementia. As the say, it runs in the family. I have been concerned about this for some time, I have had a brain ultra sound, which showed no evidence of dementia. A background of concussions can affect the test. I have had a few concussions due to playing sports. This adds to my concern, and maybe it is heightened by watching my Mom these last few months. Do I want to know, do I want my daughter to have to take care of me when I cannot? Do I want to lose all my dignity, be incontinent? No I do not.

As I read more about this gene and testing, I realized that I need more information. According to alzinfo.org, I found this information, "Research has found an increased risk for late-onset Alzheimer's in people who inherit one or two copies of a particular variation of a gene called apolipoprotein E (APOE) — the variation known as APOE e4. The finding that increased risk is linked with inheritance of the APOE e4 allele has helped explain some of the variations in age of onset of Alzheimer's disease based on whether people have inherited zero, one, or two copies of the APOE e4 allele from their parents. The more APOE e4 alleles one inherits, the lower the age of disease onset."

That was enough for me to call my health care provider and ask for an appointment with a Genetics Doctor. I now have an appointment in a few months. Now, I get to wait and agonize over the what ifs. What if I have that gene? If I have that gene, who do I tell? If I have that gene, do I agonize over this for years and years? If I have that gene, every time I forget something, do I think dementia coming to get me? If I have that gene, do I start now to plan how I want my treatment to me? If I have the gene, how do I want my ending stages to play out?

These are some of the racing thoughts and questions I ponder over.

All these questions cannot be answered right now. Maybe never answered, but I need to be prepared. I'm a planner, I want things to go as planned and when they do not I get mad. This is something I may not have any control over, but I know that I do not want my daughter to ever, and I mean ever, to go through what I'm going through. I do not want her to see her Mom slip away slowly, to have to arrange her life around my needs. My Mom did not have the knowledge we have now on dementia, her mom had a lesser form of dementia and passed away when she was 79, so her dementia never had the time to get to the stages my Mom is at. To be honest, for the first few years of my Mom's dementia we thought it was "old age". Therefore, we did not prepared like we should have.

Maybe I will go forward and be tested for the gene. I may or may not have that gene, and I may or may not get dementia. If I do have the gene, however, and they tell me it is highly likely I will get some form of dementia, I will take that information and do some soul searching. I will do things like do my will with very clear directives on signing a DNR and when to stop medication. Everyone has the right to make decisions on how they see their golden years to play out, mine will not be confused.

Is the greatest gift love, time or both?

They say the greatest gift you can give someone is love - but they also say that time heals all wounds. I agree with these statements, but loving someone is just not just saying it in an email or a text. To me, to really love someone is to be present with them.

I believe time spent with love ones is the greatest gift. For my Mom, time has no meaning. She has lost the ability to know what year, date and the actual time is. She throttles back and forth between when she was a child, to when she was in her 50's, to the present all with a 15-minute conversion with me. In the months of December, Christmas is always tomorrow, to which I gently remind her when it is. I arrive for my visits during the week same time each day at 4:05 pm, but she always asks if it is breakfast, or lunch time.

For my Mom, time is not a date on the calendar, or on a tick on a clock. It is the time spent enjoying life - the life that she has now. Time, for my mother and I, is holding her hand, talking about family members, and laughing at the Golden Girls on Sunday mornings. It is quality time. At her age, and stage of dementia, it is a balance of the good and the bad, the yin and the yang. The good is time spent with her that is is very precious, and that I know will end at some point, but hopefully not for a while. I'm a realist, however, and I know that it will be sooner than later. The bad, is that time away is stressful, wondering if she is okay, and that she is happy. Time away is time I have lost, and will never get back.

I have been spending way too much time and effort worrying and being depressed on what dementia and time has done to my Mom - I just can't let go of that feeling. But with the New Year ahead of us, for 2019 I'm determine to let that go. The time with Mom is the best time of our lives, and most importantly for myself time away from Mom is positive and productive. No more when visits are stressful and sad will I dwell on that feeling for days, I NEED TO LET THAT GO. That may be easier to write on this blog then it is in real life. We are all a work in progress, however. With the support of family & friends, and a few good beers at the bar with friends I will win this battle.

So is the greatest gift you can someone love? I say NO the greatest gift you can give anyone is time with them loving them.

Letting it GO

Let it go……

So what was your new year's resolution? Was it to be healthier, to be kinder person, to help others, to volunteer more? These are all good intentions, but for most we all fall short by mid-February.

This year I did not make a new year's resolution, instead I made a goal to live by. That is to "let it go". I was told by a few people that I need to treat myself better, not to let what's happening to my Mom get me so depressed and down. I need to "let it go". I had some time over the period between Christmas and New Year's to think a lot about this. And on Christmas was my breaking point. On Christmas Day I found myself sitting in the back seat of an Uber crying on not able to bring my Mom to my house for Christmas dinner. We did bring her dinner later that day, but I could not let go of the sadness I felt. The next few days I was away in Europe with my daughter. Normally I would be up tight, anxiety ridden, and as a good friend says, kind of bitchy. But I told myself that I will "let it go" all those feelings and enjoy the beautiful country of Ireland, and most of all enjoy my time with my daughter. Not to say that when I get tired I will be "kind of bitchy" just ask Nikki, but I did not dwell on what if's back home, I stayed present and enjoy myself.

To my surprise when I went to see my Mom the day after I got back, I showed her pictures of our trip and she asked questions about Ireland, and was very engaged. That showed me that if I keep her engaged in the present and not dwell in things I cannot changed, then we both benefit from my visits.

I'm not saying that I will not worry about Mom, and when I walk out the door forget about her, that is far from what I'm saying. What I need to do, is if she has a bad day, that I deal with her feelings right there, and not dwell on the sadness for days, I will deal with my emotions then "let it go".

In the upcoming months I have a lot of issues I need to deal with concerning her care, which I normally would worry about for days and weeks, and it would overwhelm me to point that I cannot do anything for anyone. But I will deal with what I have to do, and not let carry on for days or weeks.

Now we are not all perfect and we tend to not stay with goals or resolution's, but when and I will fall, I will pick myself up and remind myself of the goal I set and start again. I need to do this for my Mom, my family and friends that have stood by my side during my "bitchy moods", but most of all for me.

Be brave and go away alone for self-care

People often tell me to go to happy place in your head to clear your mind. I am the type of person that takes this literally. The past month or so has been pure hell for me. But, as I mentioned before, I am actively trying to "let go" of the stress and anxiety. With this current situation, however, I couldn't. With the buildup of the stress during the week, I was a mess by Friday. On top of that, I am awful for asking for help. In a passive way, I was sending out SOS to my friends. Times like these are when I am thankful that I have some great friends that come to my side when needed.

I knew I had to do something, but I did not know what, until my daughter told me she was going away alone for a weekend to do some soul searching. I thought that I could never to do that. I thought she is so brave for that. After a few beers with my friends and some good conversion, I decided that I need to go away alone and do some thinking, writing, & some affirmations to live by.

It took me about a second to figure out that I wanted to go to my happy place, which is Cape Cod. I proceeded to book a room

My first stop was my family's favorite beach. I walked the beach, talked to the seagulls, and just enjoyed the peace of the waves hitting the pier. The beach always has been a special place for me. It is very different in the winter, of course, but I found it to be especially beautiful and peaceful. It was very cold, but that did not matter to me. I kept thinking that the beach is the place that was special for my Mom. To her, it was a place that all eight of us, plus uncles, aunts and cousins would gather each summer.

I went away alone for a few reasons. I went to separate myself from what was stressing me out. I also went to strategize how I can handle all the demands on me currently. When asked if I was going to shut off my phone, I said that I could not do that. I may get a call from the nursing home. I barely answered any texts, emails or social media messages. This was very much needed.

When I'm alone, I'm far from an outgoing person. I hate small talk, which could be a self-confidence thing. I feared sitting at the bar alone, and I feared that people would think that I do not have anyone in my life to join me. I quickly realized that I don't care, I was there for me and no one else. I enjoyed sitting at the bar for my meals with a good cold beer and clam roll. Again, I did not engage in any conversion with anyone, just your friendly "Hi how are you".

As far as thinking about how to deal with my stress and demands on me… that was harder than I thought. I thought I was a strong person, for years I was the one in the family that would handle any emergencies. I always put on a brave face when adversity struck, especially when my Dad passed. I never cried and never grieved.

During my time alone I let myself ponder what is going on with my life, I said to myself, "you can't do this alone, let others help". Now I have to follow this affirmation. I hate asking for help. I've always seen it as a sign of weakness. I know this is not true, and I have plenty of people that want to help me, but I have to learn to let them, not just say, "it's okay. I will figure it out".

So, I now practice self-care, not just for me, but for my Mom, my family, my work, my volunteer work and for my friends. I would highly recommend this, if not a weekend, then maybe a day. If you think about it, how can you love others if you don't start with yourself?

Happy 87th Birthday MOM

Happy Birthday MOM!!
On March 23, 1932 Theresa Rodolfos was born to Elizabeth & Anthony Rodolfos. On March 23, 2019 Theresa (Rodolfos) Andres will turn 87 years old. Think about that for a moment - Mom has lived 762,120 hrs. 31,755 days, 1,044 months, and 8 decades. Incredible feat, I must say.

Such an accomplishment should be celebrated in a grand way, maybe throw a parade, have a big party, or go the Bruins game. It must be something big and exciting. For loved ones with dementia, this is not the appropriate way to celebrate such a wonderful day. As I have noticed over the past few years, large crowds with a lot of noise confuses my Mom. She cannot follow any of the conversions, she wants to be part of the family and even break up an argument, like she use to do in the past. Being outside the nursing home make her agitated, she thinks she is going back to her old home, or her childhood home. She is wondering where her husband, her parents, her brother & sister in law are, which all have passed.

How do you celebrate someone that has lived 762,120 hrs, 31,755 days, 1,044 months, 8 decades, and 87 years? The first thing I have learned is, don't bring up the fact she is 87 - that only reminds her that she is getting older. She asks "do I looks old?" "I moisturize my face every morning," she reminds me. "Do I have gray hair?" The best is, "well, I cannot do what the movie stars do to make them self's look younger, because everyone know what year I was born." As always, Mom is right. I do not bring it up, but I do bring up is someone special day is in March, which she asks, "What is that?" I tell her that the best Mom in the world was born March 23rd, she says, "Oh yeah, and who would that be?"

In the past few weeks Mom has been very lonely and sad, I fully understand her feeling this way. Wouldn't you be lonely and sad if you were 87 in a nursing home not surrounded by your love ones every day, only to have a visit a day for a few hours from your family? She misses her family very much. Sadly she misses her loved ones that are no longer with us. Each day, we play the game of where is her husband, her parents, her brother. The very first thing she says to me "is everyone in the family ok, don't lie to me". Even at her stage of dementia she still wants to be the caretaker of the family, she wants to nurture all of her 6 kids, 7 grandchildren, and her 10 great grandchildren. Which is definitely the most wonderful trait that my mother still has.

Again, I ask how do you celebrate someone that has lived 762,120 hrs, 31,755 days, 1,044 months, 8 decades, and 87 years? This is easy, surround her with the people that love her the most. This year like last year, we are having a dinner with just her family. This year, however, I ask that each one of us spend 1:1 quality time with our Mother, Mother-in-law, grandmother, and great-grandmother. Hold her hand, tell that you appreciate her, and tell her that she is very important part of your life, but most of all tell her you love her.

In the long winding road of life, isn't that all we want is the love of our family, and to know we play an important role in their lives.

Knowledge is power: testing for Dementia

I recently went to the Geneticist to talk about getting a test to see if I have early onset Dementia. It was the most anxiety-provoking thing I have done in years. Questions were flooding my head before my visit.

Do I really want to go?

Do I really want to know the outcome?

What do I do if I have the markers for early or late onset Dementia?

Who do I tell?

How will this affect my life going forward?

How will this affect my husband & daughter?

On and on….

I consider myself a risk taker, a "try anything" kind of gal. This is very different then agreeing to be hypnotized and being the butt of all jokes, however. It is not life or death, but it is has a heavy burden to carry the rest of your life. Many people advised me to not do it - my husband and close friends included. I took all of that in consideration. Seeing my Mom lately, and her dementia stealing the person I love made me stop and think. I realized that I don't want my daughter to go through this.

With all that, I walked into the doctor's office wanting to gain all of the knowledge I possibly can get. First, she took down all of my and my family's history with dementia, as well as the ages they presented symptoms, which is key. Then she talked about the testing, and I found out the testing for the gene is called APOE, the testing is not 100%, and it is generally for early onset dementia. With that, I was not sure if this was a waste of my time. She explained that my Mom, Grandmother, 2 uncles all had late onset dementia, and there is no testing for that. With that, however, she said that the likelihood of me getting dementia is very high, but not for about 20 years.

So with that information what can I do? She gave me some great advice. She said that when I retired to put my 401K saving into a trust, and our house in a trust. Protect any investments before 2039. Also told me to only do things that make you happy, don't waste the next 20 years doing activities that do not make you happy. She also said don't dwell in the negative, don't spend the next 20 years sitting around waiting for dementia to knock on my door. Keep active, do brain exercise like puzzles. The Dr also said I should have a long talk with my daughter about how I want to live with dementia and the possibility of her getting it. Also the biggest one, don't wait to retired at 67 or 70, if you can, retire as early as you can.

With that information, I had a mixed feeling. The chances I will not get dementia in my 60's (which is around the corner) is a good thing. Knowing there is high chance that in my late 70's is scary. She gave me some soul searching to do. What would you do? As I said I'm a risk taker, but with what I know about dementia and how it steals you from your love ones, I will not take any risks. It is a very serious subject to me.

Many thoughts, including these, have been racing in my head since my visit. I will protect my finances from the mean old Medicare (Next blog). I will not dwell on, nor will I allow myself to be dragged into any negativity. I will surround myself with only good loving people. I will not wait until the government says it ok to retire. Any work after retirement, or before, will be focus on helping caretakers of dementia patients. I will not sit around watching useless TV waiting for 2039 to come around. I will stay active and keep trying to help people. I will go to as many concerts I possibly can fit in. I will keep traveling as long as I can. These are two things I love to do.

Right now, I do not have a definite game plan. Normally I do a "to do" list to stay on track. This is different than putting together a spreadsheet for a telethon, it is my life. So, the game plan for right now in 2019 is to live life to its fullest, only let people that truly care about me in life, and treat them as a blessing. I won't dwell on things I cannot change, but I will be as accepting as I possibility can be. In a nutshell, I will live each day as a blessing, and treat people as I would want to be treated. Isn't that the golden rule of life anyway?

-Karen Vergakes NOT WAITING TO GET DEMENTIA

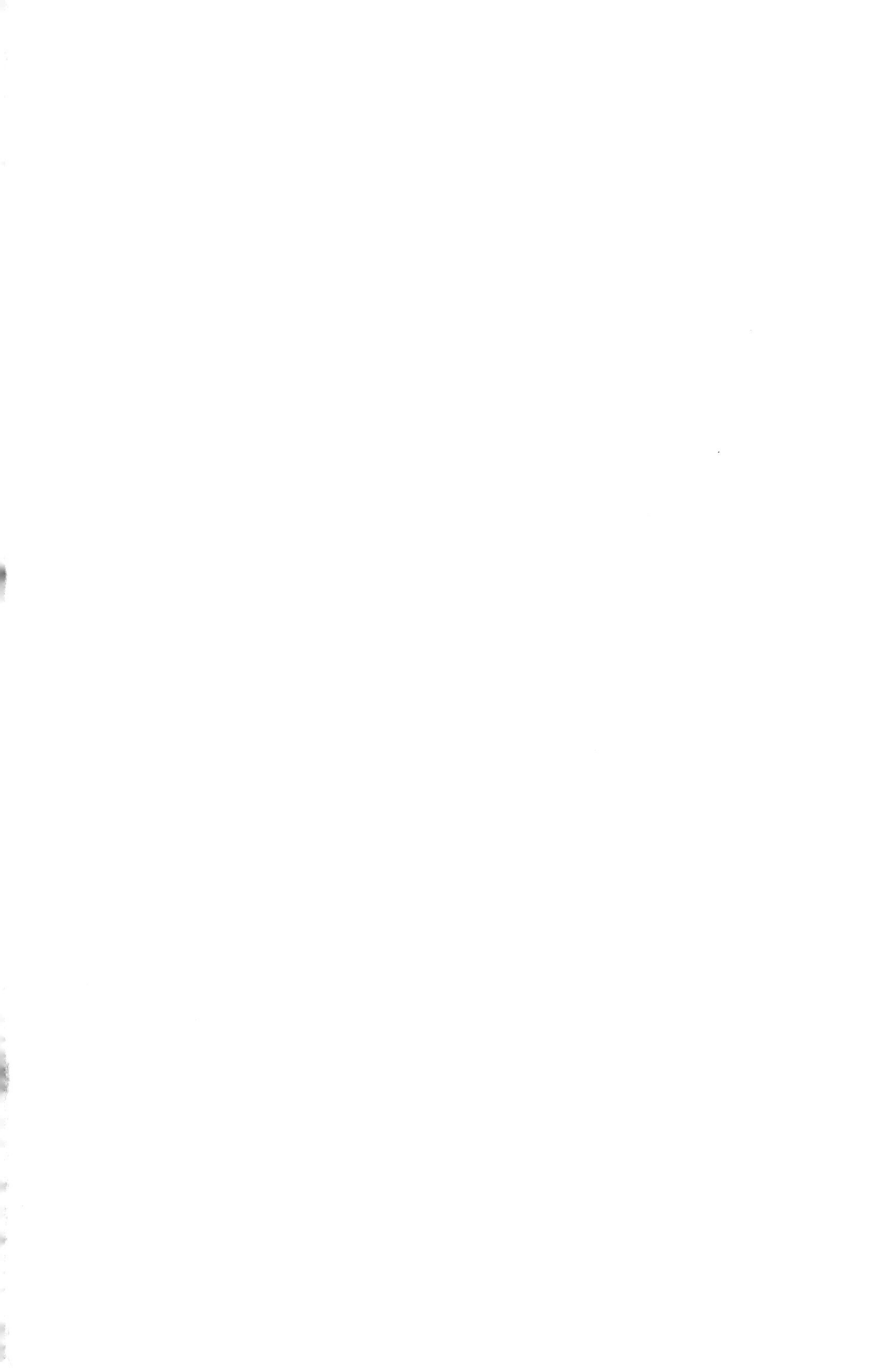

Made in the USA
Coppell, TX
15 April 2025